I0829567
1

Somatic Detox Diet

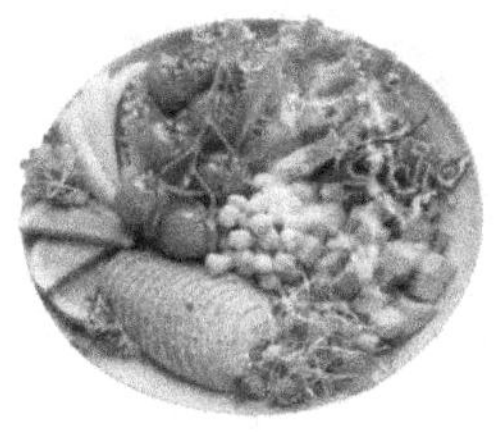

A 21-Day Cleanse to Rebalance Your Body and Mind with Simple Detox Recipes

~Sophia Wells~

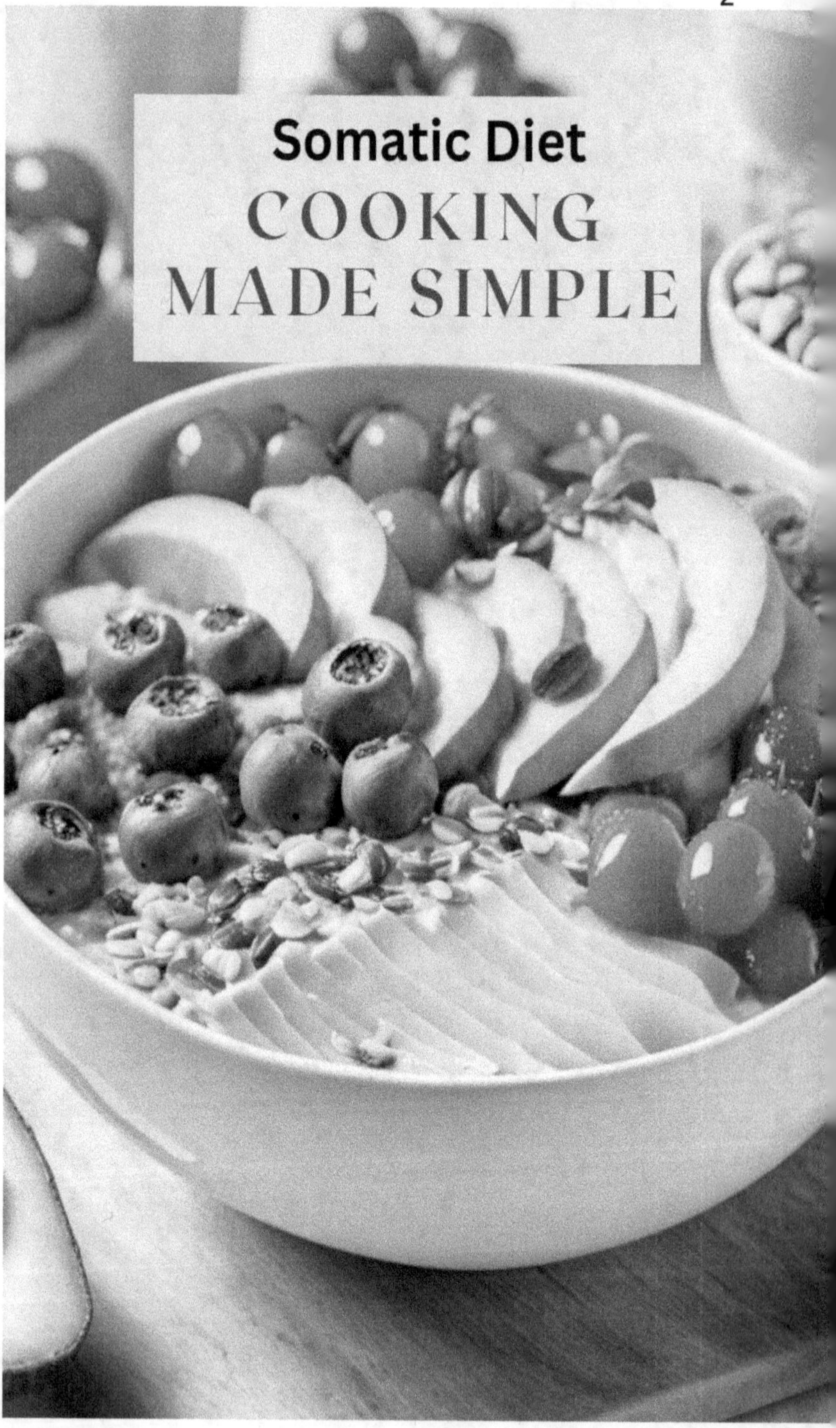

Somatic Diet
COOKING MADE SIMPLE

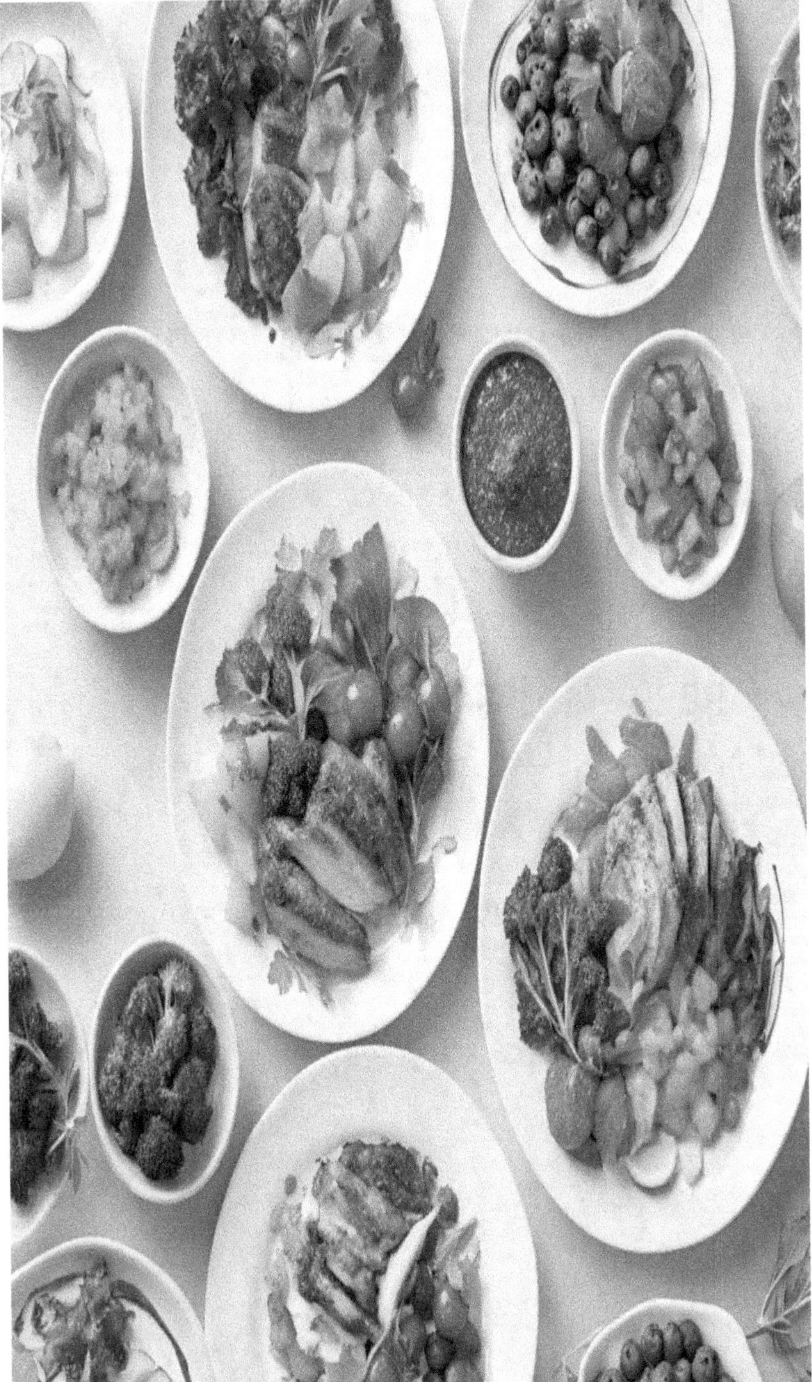

Copyright © 2024 by Sophia Wells

All rights reserved. No part of this book may be reproduced, stored in a retrieval system, or transmitted in any form or by any means—electronic, mechanical, photocopying, recording, or otherwise—without prior written permission from the publisher, except for brief quotations used in a book review.

Table of Contents

The Somatic Detox Diet Principles

Introduction

The Power of Somatic Detoxification

Hey there, health seeker! If you've picked up this book, chances are you're feeling a bit off-kilter. Maybe you're battling brain fog, struggling with unexplained aches, or just not feeling like your vibrant self. Well, let me tell you something - you're not alone. In fact, you're part of a growing tribe of folks who are waking up to the fact that our modern world, for all its wonders, can sometimes leave us feeling... well, toxic.

But here's the good news: you've just taken the first step on an incredible journey. This book isn't just another fad diet or quick fix. It's a roadmap to rediscovering your body's innate wisdom and power to heal. We're about to embark on a 21-day adventure that will transform not just your body, but your mind and spirit too.

Now, I know what you might be thinking. "Another detox plan? Been there, done that, bought the juice cleanse." But hang on a sec. This isn't about depriving yourself or following some rigid, joyless regimen. The Somatic Detox Diet is different. It's about tuning into your body, nourishing it with delicious, wholesome foods, and gently releasing the stuff that's been holding you back.

This book is for you if:

- You're tired of feeling tired all the time
- You've tried diets that left you hungry and cranky
- You're ready to break free from the cycle of cravings and crashes

- You want to feel at home in your body again
- You're curious about the connection between what you eat and how you feel
- You're looking for simple, tasty recipes that actually make you feel good

Sound familiar? Then you're in the right place, my friend.

Over the next few chapters, we're going to dive deep into the fascinating world of somatic detoxification. Don't worry if that sounds like a mouthful - we'll break it all down in plain English. You'll learn how your body and mind work together, how to stock your kitchen for success, and how to whip up meals that are both healing and delicious.

But more than that, you'll discover a new way of listening to your body. You'll learn to recognize its signals, honor its needs, and treat it with the love and respect it deserves. This isn't just about losing weight or getting clear skin (though those might be nice side effects). It's about reclaiming your vitality, your energy, and your zest for life.

So, are you ready to feel alive again? To wake up with a spring in your step and a sparkle in your eye? To rediscover the version of you that's been hiding under layers of stress and toxins?

Then let's do this thing. Turn the page, and let's start your journey to a cleaner, clearer, more vibrant you. Trust me, your future self is going to thank you for taking this step.

Welcome to the Somatic Detox Diet. Your body, mind, and spirit are in for a treat.

Chapter 1

Understanding the Mind-Body Connection

Hey there, health explorer! Ready to dive into the fascinating world of mind-body connection? Buckle up, because we're about to embark on a journey that'll change how you think about your health.

What is somatic detoxification?

Let's start with a biggie: somatic detoxification. Sounds fancy, right? But it's actually pretty simple. "Somatic" just means "relating to the body," and we all know what detoxification is. So, somatic detoxification is all about cleansing your body, but with a twist.

Unlike traditional detox methods that focus solely on the physical, somatic detoxification recognizes that your body and mind are besties. They're constantly chatting, influencing each other in ways we're only beginning to understand. This approach isn't about just cleaning out your gut or liver (though that's part of it). It's about creating harmony between your physical self and your mental state.

Think of it like this: have you ever had a stressful day and suddenly found yourself craving junk food? Or felt sluggish after a heavy meal and noticed your mood taking a nosedive? That's the mind-body connection in action, folks!

Somatic detoxification aims to break those negative cycles. We're talking about nourishing your body with foods that make you feel good physically and mentally. We're looking at practices that calm your mind and, in turn, reduce inflammation in your body. It's a holistic approach that recognizes you're not just a walking stomach or a disembodied brain – you're a complex, interconnected system.

The science behind body-mind rebalancing

Now, I know some of you might be skeptical. "Where's the proof?" you might ask. Well, science has your back on this one.

Recent studies in the field of psychoneuroimmunology (try saying that five times fast!) have shown that our thoughts and emotions can directly impact our physical health. For instance, chronic stress can lead to increased inflammation in the body, which is linked to a whole host of health issues from heart disease to depression.

But here's the cool part: it works both ways. Just as negative thoughts can harm our health, positive ones can heal. Practices like meditation and mindful eating have been shown to reduce stress hormones, lower blood pressure, and even boost our immune system.

One study published in the Journal of Psychosomatic Research found that mindfulness-based stress reduction techniques led to significant improvements in physical symptoms and quality of life for people with various health conditions. Another study in the Proceedings of the National Academy of Sciences showed that just three months of meditation practice can lead to changes in brain regions associated with learning, memory, and emotion regulation.

So when we talk about body-mind rebalancing, we're not just throwing around new-age buzzwords. We're talking about leveraging these scientific insights to create real, lasting change in your health.

How toxins affect our physical and mental well-being

Now, let's chat about toxins. And no, I'm not just talking about that questionable leftover takeout in your fridge. Our bodies are exposed to a wide range of toxins every day – from environmental pollutants to the preservatives in our food, and even the negative thoughts we harbor.

These toxins can wreak havoc on our bodies in numerous ways. They can disrupt our hormones, leading to mood swings and energy crashes. They can cause inflammation, which is linked to everything from joint pain to cognitive decline. Some toxins can even interfere with our body's ability to absorb nutrients, leaving us feeling depleted no matter how well we eat.

But here's where it gets really interesting: toxins don't just affect us physically. They can mess with our mental health too. For example, studies have found links between exposure to certain environmental toxins and increased rates of anxiety and depression. And that inflammation we talked about earlier? It's been associated with mood disorders as well.

Even the toxins we create internally through chronic stress or negative self-talk can impact our physical health. Ever noticed how you're more likely to catch a cold when you're stressed out? That's your mind-body connection at work!

The good news is, our bodies are incredible machines designed to detoxify naturally. But in our modern world, they often need a little help. That's where the Somatic Detox Diet comes in. By supporting your body's natural detoxification processes and addressing both physical and mental well-being, we can help restore balance and vitality.

So, are you starting to see how it all connects? Your mind, your body, your diet, your environment – they're all part of the same beautiful, complex system that is you. And when we approach health with this holistic mindset, amazing things can happen.

In the next chapter, we'll get practical and start preparing for your 21-day journey. But for now, take a moment to appreciate the incredible, interconnected being that you are. You've got the power to transform your health from the inside out. And trust me, this is going to be one heck of a ride!

Chapter 2

Preparing for Your 21-Day Journey

Alright, health warrior! You've got the knowledge, now it's time to prepare for action. This chapter is all about setting you up for success on your 21-day somatic detox adventure. So let's roll up our sleeves and get down to business!

Setting realistic goals and expectations

First things first — let's talk about goals. Now, I know you might be dreaming of dropping 20 pounds or achieving zen-like enlightenment in just three weeks. And while I love your enthusiasm, let's keep it real.

The Somatic Detox Diet isn't about quick fixes or miracle cures. It's about creating sustainable changes that'll benefit you long after these 21 days are over. So, let's set some achievable, meaningful goals:

1. Improved energy levels: Imagine waking up feeling refreshed, not reaching for that third cup of coffee by 2 PM.

2. Better digestion: Less bloating, more regularity (yeah, we're going there!).

3. Clearer skin: Your largest organ often reflects what's going on inside.

4. Improved mood stability: Less irritability, more calm.

5. Reduced cravings: Saying goodbye to those 3 AM cookie raids.

Remember, everyone's journey is unique. You might see dramatic changes in some areas and subtle shifts in others. The key is to listen to your body and celebrate every win, no matter how small.

Now, a word on weight loss. While many people do shed some pounds on this plan, that's not our primary goal. We're after deep, cellular health here. So if the scale doesn't budge but you're feeling energized and vibrant, that's a massive win in my book!

Creating a supportive environment

You know that saying, "You are the average of the five people you spend the most time with"? Well, it applies to health too. Your environment plays a huge role in your success, so let's make it work for you:

1. Communicate with your loved ones: Let them know what you're doing and why it's important to you. You might even inspire them to join in!

2. Clear out temptations: Do a pantry purge. Donate or toss out foods that don't align with your new goals. Out of sight, out of mind!

3. Set up your space for success: Create a designated area for meal prep, stock up on glass containers for leftovers, maybe even set up a small meditation corner.

4. Plan for social situations:
Eating out or attending events doesn't have to derail you. Have a game plan – maybe eat a small meal before, or scope out menu options in advance.

5. Find an accountability buddy:
Whether it's a friend, family member, or an online community, having support can make all the difference.

Remember, you're not just changing your diet – you're shifting your lifestyle. Make your environment reflect the healthy, vibrant person you're becoming.

Stocking your kitchen with detox-friendly ingredients

Now for the fun part – shopping! Your kitchen is about to become your health headquarters. Here's what you'll want to stock up on:

1. Leafy greens: Kale, spinach, arugula, Swiss chard. These are detox superstars, packed with chlorophyll to support liver function.

2. Cruciferous veggies: Broccoli, cauliflower, Brussels sprouts. They're rich in compounds that support detoxification pathways.

3. Berries: Blueberries, strawberries, raspberries. Antioxidant powerhouses that fight free radicals.

4. Herbs and spices: Turmeric, ginger, garlic, cilantro. These aren't just flavor boosters – they have potent anti-inflammatory properties.

5. Healthy fats: Avocados, olive oil, nuts, and seeds. They help absorb fat-soluble vitamins and keep you feeling satisfied.

6. Lean proteins: Wild-caught fish, organic chicken, legumes. Protein is crucial for supporting detox pathways and maintaining muscle mass.

7. Whole grains: Quinoa, brown rice, oats. They provide fiber and sustained energy.

8. Fermented foods: Sauerkraut, kimchi, kefir. These probiotic-rich foods support gut health, which is key to overall well-being.

9. Detox-supporting teas: Green tea, dandelion root, milk thistle. These can give your liver an extra boost.

10. Filtered water: Hydration is crucial for flushing out toxins. Invest in a good water filter if you can.

Pro tip: Buy organic when possible, especially for the "Dirty Dozen" (foods most likely to have pesticide residues). Your body will thank you! **As you stock up,** remember – this isn't about deprivation. It's about nourishing your body with high-quality, nutrient-dense foods that'll make you feel amazing.

So there you have it, friend! You're all set to embark on this transformative journey. Remember, preparation is key, but don't get hung up on perfection. This is about progress, not perfection. You've got this!

In the next chapter, we'll dive into the core principles of the Somatic Detox Diet. Get ready to revolutionize your relationship with food and your body. Exciting times ahead!

Chapter 3

The Somatic Detox Diet Principles

Alright, nutrition enthusiast! You've set your goals, prepped your environment, and stocked your kitchen. Now it's time to dive into the meat and potatoes (or should I say kale and quinoa?) of the Somatic Detox Diet. Let's unpack the principles that'll guide you through this transformative journey.

Key nutrients for detoxification

Your body is a natural detoxification machine, but like any good machine, it needs the right fuel to run smoothly. Here are the star players in the detox game:

1. Glutathione: Often called the "master antioxidant," glutathione is crucial for liver detoxification. Foods rich in sulfur like garlic, onions, and cruciferous veggies help boost glutathione production.

2. B Vitamins: These little powerhouses support various detox pathways. Load up on leafy greens, whole grains, and nutritional yeast.

3. Vitamin C: This antioxidant superhero helps neutralize free radicals and supports the immune system. Citrus fruits, berries, and bell peppers are great sources.

4. Magnesium: Essential for hundreds of biochemical reactions, including detox processes. Find it in dark chocolate, almonds, and spinach.

5. Omega-3 fatty acids: These anti-inflammatory fats support brain health and detoxification.

Wild-caught fatty fish, chia seeds, and walnuts are excellent sources.

6. Fiber: It's not glamorous, but fiber is crucial for binding to toxins and escorting them out of your body. Aim for a mix of soluble (oats, apples) and insoluble (whole grains, veggie skins) fiber.

Remember, these nutrients work synergistically. It's not about mega-dosing on any one thing, but rather creating a diverse, nutrient-dense diet.

Foods to embrace and avoid

Now, let's talk about what should and shouldn't be on your plate:

Embrace:

- **Leafy greens:** Spinach, kale, Swiss chard – the more, the merrier!

- **Cruciferous veggies:** Broccoli, cauliflower, Brussels sprouts are detox dynamos.

- **Berries:** Nature's candy, packed with antioxidants.

- **Herbs and spices:** Turmeric, ginger, cilantro – flavor and healing in one package.

- **Clean proteins:** Wild-caught fish, organic poultry, legumes, and plant-based proteins.

- **Healthy fats:** Avocados, olive oil, nuts, and seeds.
- **Fermented foods:** Kimchi, sauerkraut, kefir for gut health.
- **Green tea:** Loaded with catechins that support liver function.

Avoid (or significantly reduce):
- **Processed foods:** If it comes in a box with a long ingredient list, it's probably best to skip it.
- **Refined sugar:** It's inflammatory and can disrupt your hormones.
- **Alcohol:** Your liver has enough to do without this extra burden.

- **Caffeine:** A little green tea is fine, but skip the energy drinks and excessive coffee.

- **Conventional dairy:** If you tolerate dairy, opt for organic, grass-fed sources.

- **Gluten:** Many people find they feel better without it, at least during the detox period.

- **Artificial additives:** Colors, flavors, sweeteners – your body doesn't need these.

Remember, this isn't about perfection. If you slip up, don't stress. Just get back on track with your next meal.

Balancing macronutrients for optimal results

You've probably heard of macronutrients – proteins, fats, and carbohydrates. But did you know that balancing these can significantly impact your detox journey? **Let's break it down:**

Proteins (20-30% of calories): Protein is crucial for supporting detox pathways and maintaining muscle mass. Opt for clean sources like wild-caught fish, organic poultry, eggs, legumes, and plant-based proteins. Aim for about 0.8-1 gram of protein per kilogram of body weight.

Fats (30-40% of calories):

Don't fear fat! Healthy fats are essential for hormone balance, nutrient absorption, and feeling satisfied. Focus on sources like avocados, olive oil, nuts, seeds, and fatty fish rich in omega-3s.

Carbohydrates (30-50% of calories):

Carbs aren't the enemy, but choose wisely. Opt for complex carbs from vegetables, fruits, and whole grains. These provide fiber for detoxification and steady energy without blood sugar spikes.

Here's a pro tip: Think of your plate as a pie chart. Half should be colorful veggies, a quarter lean protein, and a quarter complex carbs, with a thumb-sized portion of healthy fats.

Remember, these percentages are guidelines, not strict rules. Some people feel best with more protein, others with more carbs. Listen to your body and adjust accordingly.

Hydration: The unsung hero

We can't talk about detox without mentioning water. Aim for at least 8 glasses a day, more if you're active. Herbal teas and infused water count too. Proper hydration helps flush toxins, supports kidney function, and can even help with cravings.

A word on portion sizes

While we're not counting calories on this plan, portion control still matters. Use your hand as a guide:
- **Protein:** Palm-sized portion
- **Veggies:** As much as you can fit in two open hands

- **Complex carbs:** Cupped hand portion
- **Fats:** Thumb-sized portion

This method is portable and personalized – perfect for our on-the-go lives!

Remember, the Somatic Detox Diet isn't about restriction – it's about nourishment. We're flooding your body with nutrients, supporting its natural detox processes, and creating an environment for healing and vitality.

In the next chapter, we'll dive into Week One of your journey, complete with meal plans and recipes. Get ready to feel the difference that mindful, nourishing eating can make. Your body is about to thank you in ways you never imagined!

Chapter 4

<u>Week One - Gentle Cleansing (Days 1-7)</u>

Welcome to Week One of your Somatic Detox journey! This week is all about easing into the process, allowing your body to adjust gradually. We'll focus on gentle cleansing, introducing nourishing foods, and establishing mindful practices. Let's dive in!

Before diving further, if you find value in what you've read so far, I'd be grateful if you left a review. Your thoughts not only guide other readers but also help ensure the book reaches those who may benefit from it. Your support means a lot!

Daily meal plans and recipes

I'll provide a sample day's meal plan, and then we'll explore some delicious, detox-friendly recipes. Remember, listen to your body and adjust portions as needed.

Sample Day:

Breakfast: Green Goddess Smoothie

Snack: Apple slices with almond butter

Lunch: Cleansing Lentil Soup

Snack: Cucumber rounds with hummus

Dinner: Baked salmon with roasted vegetables and quinoa

Now, let's get cooking! Here are some easy, nutrient-packed recipes to kickstart your detox:

1. Green Goddess Smoothie

Ingredients:
- 1 cup spinach
- 1/2 avocado
- 1 banana
- 1 tbsp chia seeds
- 1 cup unsweetened almond milk
- 1/2 tsp spirulina (optional)

Blend all ingredients until smooth. This powerhouse smoothie is packed with fiber, healthy fats, and chlorophyll to support detoxification.

2. Cleansing Lentil Soup
Ingredients:
- 1 cup red lentils
- 1 diced onion
- 2 minced garlic cloves
- 1 diced carrot
- 1 tsp turmeric
- 1 tsp cumin
- 4 cups vegetable broth
- Juice of 1 lemon

- Salt and pepper to taste

Sauté onion and garlic. Add spices, lentils, carrot, and broth. Simmer for 20 minutes. Blend if desired. Add lemon juice before serving.

3. Baked Salmon with Roasted Vegetables

Ingredients:

- 4 oz wild-caught salmon
- 1 cup mixed vegetables (broccoli, cauliflower, Brussels sprouts)
- 1 tbsp olive oil
- 1 tsp herbs de Provence
- Salt and pepper to taste

Preheat the oven to 400°F. Toss veggies with olive oil and herbs. Bake for 20 minutes. Add salmon to the pan and bake for another 12-15 minutes.

Mindful eating practices

Mindful eating is a crucial part of the Somatic Detox Diet. It's not just about what you eat, but how you eat. Here are some practices to incorporate:

1. Eat without distractions: Turn off the TV, put away your phone, and focus on your meal.

2. Chew thoroughly: Aim for 20-30 chews per bite. This aids digestion and helps you eat more slowly.

3. Practice gratitude: Before eating, take a moment to appreciate your food and those who helped bring it to your plate.

4. Use all your senses: Notice the colors, smells, textures, and flavors of your food.

5. Listen to your body: Eat when you're hungry, stop when you're satisfied (not stuffed).

6. Breathe: Take a few deep breaths before meals to activate your parasympathetic nervous system, which aids digestion.

Try implementing one or two of these practices this week. As they become habits, add more.

Gentle exercise routines to support detoxification

Exercise is a fantastic way to support your body's natural detox processes. It boosts circulation, promotes lymphatic drainage, and helps you sweat out toxins. But remember, we're going gently this week. Here are some ideas:

1. Morning stretch routine (10-15 minutes):

- Cat-Cow pose (5 rounds)
- Downward Dog to Forward Fold (5 rounds)
- Gentle twists (hold for 30 seconds each side)
- Child's Pose (hold for 1 minute)

2. Afternoon walk (20-30 minutes):

A brisk walk in nature can do wonders for your physical and

mental health. Aim for 20-30 minutes, but listen to your body.

3. Evening yoga flow (15-20 minutes):

- Sun Salutations (3 rounds)
- Warrior I and II poses (hold for 30 seconds each side)
- Triangle pose (hold for 30 seconds each side)
- Legs up the wall pose (hold for 5 minutes)

4. Rebounding (5-10 minutes):

If you have access to a mini-trampoline, gentle bouncing is great for lymphatic drainage. Start with just a few minutes and build up.

5. Deep breathing exercises (5 minutes, anytime):
Try box breathing: Inhale for 4 counts, hold for 4, exhale for 4, hold for 4. Repeat for 5 minutes.

Remember, the goal is to move your body gently, not to push yourself to exhaustion. If you're feeling tired, it's okay to take a rest day.

As you progress through this first week, pay attention to how your body feels. You might experience some mild detox symptoms like headaches or fatigue. This is normal as your body adjusts. Stay hydrated and rest when you need to.

Celebrate every small victory - maybe you drank more water today, or you tried a new vegetable. These small steps add up to big changes over time.

In the next chapter, we'll ramp things up a bit as we move into Week Two. But for now, focus on establishing these new habits and nourishing your body with wholesome foods and gentle movement.

Remember, you're not just changing your diet - you're embarking on a journey of self-discovery and healing. Be patient and kind with yourself. You've got this!

Chapter 5

Week Two - Deep Cleansing (Days 8-14)

Welcome to Week Two, detox warrior! You've made it through the gentle introduction, and now it's time to kick things up a notch. This week, we're diving deeper into the cleansing process, targeting those stubborn toxins, and amping up our stress-reduction game. Ready? Let's go!

Intensifying the detox process

As your body has adjusted to the new eating patterns, we can now intensify the detox process. Here's how:

1. Increase hydration: Aim for 10-12 glasses of water daily. Try starting your day with warm lemon water to stimulate digestion and support liver function.

2. Amp up the greens: Introduce more bitter greens like dandelion and arugula. These stimulate bile production, aiding in toxin elimination.

3. Dry brushing: Before showering, spend 5 minutes dry brushing your skin. This stimulates lymphatic drainage and helps shed dead skin cells.

4. Intermittent fasting: If it feels right for you, try a 12-14 hour overnight fast. For example, finish dinner by 7 PM and have breakfast at 7-9 AM the next day.

5. Sweat it out: Increase your exercise intensity slightly, or try a sauna session if available. Sweating is a great way to eliminate toxins through the skin.

Remember, listen to your body. If any of these feel too intense, dial it back. This isn't about pushing yourself to extremes.

Recipes for eliminating stubborn toxins

Let's explore some potent recipes designed to support your body's detox pathways:

1. Liver-Loving Beet Juice

Ingredients:

- 1 medium beet

- 2 carrots

- 1 apple

- 1-inch piece of ginger
- 1/2 lemon, juiced

Juice all ingredients and enjoy immediately. Beets are fantastic for supporting liver function, while ginger aids digestion and reduces inflammation.

2. Detox Broth

Ingredients:
- 8 cups water
- 1 onion, quartered
- 2 garlic cloves, crushed
- 1-inch piece of ginger, sliced
- 1 cup chopped celery
- 1 cup chopped carrots

- 1/2 cup chopped parsley
- 1 tbsp apple cider vinegar
- 1 tsp turmeric
- Sea salt to taste

Simmer all ingredients for 1-2 hours. Strain and sip throughout the day. This nutrient-dense broth supports hydration and provides essential minerals.

3. Cleansing Kitchari

Ingredients:
- 1/2 cup mung beans, soaked overnight
- 1/2 cup basmati rice
- 1 tbsp coconut oil

- 1 tsp cumin seeds
- 1 tsp mustard seeds
- 1 tsp turmeric
- 1-inch piece of ginger, grated
- 2 cups mixed vegetables (carrots, zucchini, leafy greens)
- 4 cups water
- Salt to taste

Rinse mung beans and rice. In a pot, heat oil and add seeds. When they pop, add turmeric and ginger. Add beans, rice, and water. Simmer for 20 minutes, then add vegetables and cook until tender. This Ayurvedic dish is easy to digest and supports detoxification.

Incorporating stress-reduction techniques

Stress can hinder detoxification, so let's focus on some powerful stress-reduction techniques:

1. Progressive Muscle Relaxation (PMR):

Lie down comfortably. Starting from your toes, tense each muscle group for 5 seconds, then relax for 10 seconds. Work your way up to your face. This practice helps release physical tension and calms the mind.

2. 4-7-8 Breathing: Inhale for 4 counts, hold for 7, exhale for 8.

Repeat 4 times. This technique activates the parasympathetic nervous system, promoting relaxation.

3. Mindfulness Meditation:
Start with just 5 minutes a day. Sit comfortably, focus on your breath, and when your mind wanders (it will!), gently bring it back to your breath. This practice can reduce cortisol levels and improve overall well-being.

4. Nature Bathing:
Spend 20 minutes in nature daily. Whether it's a park, your backyard,

or a nearby trail, connecting with nature can significantly reduce stress hormones.

5. Journaling:

Before bed, write down three things you're grateful for and any thoughts or feelings you want to release. This can help clear your mind and improve sleep quality.

6. Epsom Salt Bath:

Twice this week, take a warm bath with 2 cups of Epsom salts. The magnesium in the salts can help relax muscles and support detoxification.

As you move through this week, you might notice some interesting changes. Perhaps your energy levels are fluctuating, or you're experiencing vivid dreams. You might feel emotional or have some skin breakouts. These are all normal signs that your body is detoxifying. Stay hydrated, rest when you need to, and trust the process.

Remember, detoxification isn't just about eliminating physical toxins. It's also about releasing mental and emotional "toxins" - negative thought patterns, stress, and limiting beliefs. Be gentle with yourself as you navigate this process.

Celebrate your progress! You're halfway through the program, and you're doing amazing work for your health. In the next chapter, we'll start focusing on rebalancing and preparing for life beyond the 21 days.

Keep going, detox champion! Your body and mind are thanking you for this incredible gift of health and self-care.

Chapter 6

Week Three - Rebalancing and Rejuvenation (Days 15-21)

Congratulations, health champion! You've made it to the final week of your Somatic Detox journey. This week is all about consolidating the gains you've made and preparing for a sustainable, vibrant future. Let's dive into how we can make this lifestyle stick for the long haul!

Transitioning to a sustainable lifestyle

The goal isn't to stay on a strict detox forever - it's to create habits that support your health for life. Here's how to make the transition:

1. Gradual reintroduction: Slowly reintroduce foods you've been avoiding, one at a time. Pay attention to how your body reacts. This helps identify any sensitivities you may have developed.

2. 80/20 rule: Aim to eat detox-friendly foods 80% of the time, allowing for more flexibility with the other 20%. This balance keeps things sustainable without sacrificing your health goals.

3. Meal prep: Set aside time each week to prepare healthy meals. This makes it easier to stick to your new habits when life gets busy.

4. Create a support system: Share your journey with friends or family. Having support can make a huge difference in maintaining your new lifestyle.

5. Regular check-ins: Schedule monthly "health check-ins" with yourself. How are you feeling?

What's working? What isn't? Adjust as needed.

Remember, this isn't about perfection - it's about progress. Small, consistent choices add up to big changes over time.

Nutrient-dense recipes for long-term health

Let's explore some delicious, nutrient-packed recipes that will keep you feeling great long after the detox ends:

1. Rainbow Quinoa Bowl
Ingredients:
- 1 cup cooked quinoa

- 1/4 cup each of diced red pepper, yellow pepper, and cucumber
- 1/4 avocado, sliced
- 1/4 cup chickpeas
- Handful of spinach
- 2 tbsp pumpkin seeds
- Dressing: 1 tbsp olive oil, 1 tsp lemon juice, pinch of salt and pepper

Arrange all ingredients in a bowl and drizzle with dressing. This colorful bowl provides a wide range of nutrients and can be easily customized.

2. Omega-Boost Smoothie

Ingredients:

- 1 cup unsweetened almond milk

- 1 tbsp ground flaxseed
- 1 tbsp chia seeds
- 1/2 cup frozen blueberries
- 1 handful spinach
- 1/2 banana
- 1 scoop plant-based protein powder (optional)

Blend all ingredients until smooth. This smoothie is packed with omega-3 fatty acids, fiber, and antioxidants.

3. Herb-Crusted Baked Cod

Ingredients:
- 4 oz cod filet
- 1 tbsp almond flour

- 1 tbsp chopped fresh herbs
(parsley, dill, basil)
- 1 tsp lemon zest
- 1 tbsp olive oil
- Salt and pepper to taste

Mix almond flour, herbs, and lemon zest. Brush cod with olive oil, coat with herb mixture. Bake at 400°F for 12-15 minutes. Serve with roasted vegetables and quinoa for a complete meal.

Mindfulness practices for emotional balance

Emotional wellbeing is just as important as physical health. Here are some practices to incorporate for long-term emotional balance:

1. Daily gratitude practice: Each morning, write down three things you're grateful for. This simple act can shift your focus to the positive aspects of your life.

2. Loving-kindness meditation: Spend 5-10 minutes daily sending loving thoughts to yourself and others. Start with "May I be happy, may I be healthy, may I be safe, may

I live with ease." Then extend these wishes to loved ones, neutral people, and even those you find difficult.

3. Body scan: Once a day, lie down and mentally scan your body from toes to head, noticing any sensations without judgment. This practice increases body awareness and can help you identify and release tension.

4. Mindful movement: Incorporate mindful movement like yoga or tai chi into your routine. These practices combine physical activity with mindfulness, promoting both physical and emotional balance.

5. Emotion journaling: When you experience strong emotions, take a moment to write about them. What triggered the emotion? How does it feel in your body? This can help you process emotions more effectively.

6. Digital detox: Set aside time each day to disconnect from devices. Use this time to connect with nature, loved ones, or yourself.

7. Boundaries practice: Learn to set and maintain healthy boundaries.

This might mean saying no to commitments that don't align with your values or limiting time with people who drain your energy.

As you move through this final week, reflect on how far you've come. Notice the changes in your energy levels, your mood, your sleep quality. Celebrate these victories, no matter how small they might seem.

Remember, health is a journey, not a destination. There will be ups and downs, and that's okay. What matters is that you're making conscious choices to support your wellbeing.

As we wrap up this 21-day journey, I want you to know how proud you should be of yourself. You've taken a significant step towards better health and self-awareness. But this isn't the end - it's just the beginning of your new, vibrant life.

In the next chapter, we'll discuss how to maintain your results and handle potential challenges that may arise. You've laid a strong foundation - now let's make sure it lasts a lifetime!

Keep shining, healthy warrior.

The best is yet to come!

Chapter 7

Beyond the 21 Days - Maintaining Your Results

Congratulations, wellness warrior! You've completed the 21-day Somatic Detox, but your journey to vibrant health is just beginning. This chapter is all about keeping that detox glow alive and thriving in the real world. Let's dive into how you can make this lifestyle stick for the long haul!

Integrating detox principles into daily life

1. Morning Ritual: Start your day with a glass of warm lemon water. This simple habit supports hydration, digestion, and gentle detoxification.

2. Eat the Rainbow: Aim to include a variety of colorful fruits and vegetables in your meals. Each color represents different phytonutrients that support various aspects of health.

3. Mindful Eating: Continue practicing mindful eating. Take a few deep breaths before meals, chew thoroughly, and pay attention to your body's hunger and fullness cues.

4. Stay Hydrated: Keep that water bottle handy! Aim for half your body weight in ounces of water daily. Herbal teas count too!

5. Regular Movement: Find ways to move your body that you enjoy. Whether it's yoga, dancing, hiking, or swimming, consistent movement supports detoxification and overall wellbeing.

6. Dry Brushing: Incorporate dry brushing into your shower routine 2-3 times a week to support lymphatic drainage and skin health.

7. Digital Detox: Set aside time each day to unplug from devices. This mental detox is just as important as the physical one!

Remember, it's not about perfection. If you slip up, don't beat yourself up. Just get back on track with your next meal or next day.

Strategies for handling social situations and travel

Social events and travel can be challenging when you're trying to maintain a healthy lifestyle. Here are some strategies to help you navigate these situations:

1. Eat Before You Go: Have a small, nutrient-dense snack before heading to social events. This can help curb hunger and reduce the temptation to overindulge.

2. BYO Healthy Option: When possible, bring a healthy dish to share. This ensures you'll have at least one detox-friendly option.

3. Stay Hydrated: Alternate alcoholic drinks with water. This helps you stay hydrated and can reduce overall alcohol consumption.

4. Practice the Plate Method: Fill half your plate with veggies, a quarter with lean protein, and a quarter with complex carbs. This works at restaurants, buffets, or dinner parties.

5. Travel Smart: Pack healthy snacks like nuts, seeds, and fresh fruit for trips. Research healthy restaurant options at your destination in advance.

6. Hotel Hacks: Request a mini-fridge in your hotel room to store healthy snacks and breakfast items. Pack a travel blender for on-the-go smoothies.

7. Maintain Sleep Routine: As much as possible, stick to your regular sleep schedule. Good sleep supports detoxification and helps manage stress.

8. Move Daily: Even if you can't maintain your regular exercise routine, find ways to move. Take a walk, do some hotel room yoga, or try bodyweight exercises.

Remember, it's about balance. Enjoy special meals or treats occasionally without guilt. It's what you do most of the time that counts.

Seasonal mini-cleanses for ongoing wellness

Incorporating shorter detox periods throughout the year can help you reset and maintain your wellness goals. Here are some ideas for seasonal mini-cleanses:

Spring Renewal (3-5 days):

- Focus on bitter greens like dandelion and arugula to support liver detoxification.

- Try a gentle juice cleanse or increase your intake of fresh, seasonal produce.

- Practice oil pulling each morning to support oral health and detoxification.

Summer Hydration Boost (3-5 days):

- Increase water intake and enjoy hydrating foods like watermelon and cucumber.

- Try a fruit and vegetable-based smoothie cleanse.
- Practice contrast showers (alternating hot and cold) to boost circulation.

Fall Immune Support (3-5 days):
- Focus on warming, immune-boosting foods like ginger, garlic, and mushrooms.
- Try an Ayurvedic kitchari cleanse to support digestion.
- Practice daily dry brushing to support lymphatic health.

Winter Restoration (3-5 days):
- Emphasize nourishing soups and broths.

- Try an elimination diet to identify any food sensitivities.
- Practice restorative yoga and meditation to support mental detoxification.

During these mini-cleanses, revisit the principles and recipes from your 21-day detox. Use this time to check in with your body, reset any habits that might have slipped, and recommit to your health goals.

Remember, these mini-cleanses are meant to support your ongoing wellness journey, not to be a drastic departure from your regular healthy lifestyle. Always listen to your body and adjust as needed.

As you continue on your wellness journey, remember that health is not a destination—it's a lifelong adventure. There will be ups and downs, challenges and triumphs. The key is to stay connected to your 'why'—the reason you embarked on this journey in the first place.

Celebrate your successes, learn from your setbacks, and above all, be kind to yourself. You're doing amazing work in taking charge of your health and wellbeing.

In the next chapter, we'll address some common challenges and FAQs to help you troubleshoot any issues that might arise. Remember, you've got this! Your body is thanking you for this incredible gift of health and self-care. Keep shining, wellness warrior!

Chapter 8

Troubleshooting and FAQs

Welcome to the troubleshooting chapter, health explorer! Even the smoothest journeys have a few bumps along the way. This chapter is all about addressing common challenges, adjusting the plan for specific needs, and knowing when to call in the pros. Let's dive in and tackle those tricky situations head-on!

Common challenges and how to overcome them

1. Challenge: Intense cravings

Solution: Cravings are often your body's way of communicating. Try these strategies:

- **Hydrate:** Sometimes thirst masquerades as hunger.

- **Eat a balanced snack:** Combine protein, healthy fat, and complex carbs.

- **Distract yourself:** Go for a walk or call a friend.

- **Mindfulness:** Observe the craving without judgment. It will often pass.

2. Challenge: Low energy

Solution: Energy dips are common during detox. Here's how to boost your vitality:

- **Ensure adequate calorie intake:** You might need more fuel than you think.

- **Balance blood sugar:** Include protein and healthy fats with each meal.

- **Power nap:** A 20-minute nap can work wonders.

- **Gentle exercise:** A short walk can energize you.

3. Challenge: Digestive discomfort
Solution: Your gut might need time to adjust. Try these tips:

- **Chew thoroughly:** This aids digestion and nutrient absorption.
- **Incorporate fermented foods:** They support gut health.
- **Try digestive enzymes:** Consult your healthcare provider first.
- **Stay hydrated:** Water helps move things along.

4. Challenge: Difficulty sleeping
Solution: Good sleep is crucial for detoxification. Here's how to improve it:
- **Stick to a sleep schedule:** Even on weekends.

- **Create a bedtime routine:** This signals your body it's time to wind down.
- **Limit screen time:** The blue light can disrupt sleep hormones.
- **Try a magnesium supplement:** It can promote relaxation (consult your doctor first).

5. **Challenge:** Social pressure
Solution: Staying on track in social situations can be tough. Try these strategies:
- **Communicate your goals:** Let friends and family know what you're doing and why.

- **Suggest health-friendly activities:** Propose a hike instead of happy hour.
- **Prepare responses:** Have a polite "no thank you" ready for food pushers.
- **Focus on connection:** Remember, socializing is about people, not just food.

Adjusting the plan for specific health conditions

While the Somatic Detox Diet is designed to be gentle and nourishing, some health conditions may require modifications. Always consult with your healthcare provider before starting any new diet or exercise program, especially if you have a pre-existing condition.

1. Diabetes:

- Monitor blood sugar closely, especially in the first week.
- Emphasize low-glycemic foods and complex carbohydrates.
- Include protein with each meal to stabilize blood sugar.

2. Heart disease:

- Focus on heart-healthy fats like omega-3s.
- Limit sodium intake.

- Incorporate more potassium-rich foods like bananas and sweet potatoes.

3. Kidney disease:

- Adjust protein intake based on your doctor's recommendations.
- Monitor potassium and phosphorus intake.
- Stay hydrated, but don't overdo it – follow your doctor's fluid guidelines.

4. Autoimmune conditions:

- Consider an autoimmune protocol (AIP) version of the detox.

- Pay extra attention to gut health with probiotic-rich foods.
- Emphasize anti-inflammatory foods like turmeric and ginger.

5. Pregnancy or breastfeeding:

- Avoid any fasting or calorie restriction.
- Focus on nutrient-dense foods rather than elimination.
- Ensure adequate protein and healthy fat intake.

Remember, these are general guidelines. Your specific needs may vary, which is why professional guidance is crucial.

When to seek professional guidance

While this program is designed to be safe for most people, there are times when you should consult a healthcare professional:

1. Persistent symptoms: If you experience ongoing fatigue, digestive issues, or other concerning symptoms that don't improve after the first week, it's time to check in with a doctor.

2. Chronic health conditions: If you have any pre-existing health conditions, consult your healthcare provider before starting the detox and throughout the process.

3. Medication interactions: Some foods can interact with medications. If you're on any prescriptions, talk to your doctor or pharmacist about potential interactions.

4. Extreme weight loss or gain: While some weight fluctuation is normal during a detox, significant changes should be discussed with a healthcare provider.

5. Severe mood changes: If you experience persistent low mood or anxiety, reach out to a mental health professional.

6. Pregnancy or breastfeeding: These are special times nutritionally. Always consult with your OB/GYN or midwife before making dietary changes.

7. Eating disorder history: If you have a history of disordered eating, work with a registered dietitian to ensure this program is appropriate and safe for you.

8. Athletic performance: If you're an athlete, consult with a sports nutritionist to ensure the detox meets your specific needs.

Remember, seeking help isn't a sign of weakness – it's a smart way to ensure you're getting the most out of your health journey while staying safe.

FAQs

Q: Can I exercise during the detox?
A: Absolutely! But listen to your body. Gentle exercises like yoga, walking, and swimming are great. If you feel overly fatigued, scale back.

Q: I'm always hungry. Am I doing something wrong?

A: You shouldn't feel starved. Try increasing your portion sizes, especially with vegetables and lean proteins. Also, ensure you're staying hydrated.

Q: Can I drink coffee during the detox?

A: We recommend avoiding coffee for the 21 days. If you're a regular coffee drinker, taper off gradually to avoid withdrawal headaches. Green tea can be a good alternative.

Q: I'm not seeing results. Should I quit?

A: Remember, everyone's body responds differently. Focus on how you feel rather than just physical changes. If you have concerns, consult with a healthcare provider.

Q: Can I do this detox long-term?

A: The 21-day program is designed as a reset. For long-term health, transition to a balanced, whole-food diet using the principles you've learned.

Remember, your body is unique, and your journey will be too. It's okay to adapt the program to fit your needs, as long as you're staying true to the core principles of nourishing your body with whole, nutrient-dense foods.

You've got this, health champion! In our final chapter, we'll wrap up with some inspiring success stories and final words of encouragement. Keep going – your vibrant, healthier self is just around the corner!

Chapter 9

The Somatic Detox Recipe Collection

Welcome to the heart of our Somatic Detox journey - the recipe collection! This chapter is your go-to resource for delicious, nourishing meals that support your body's natural detoxification processes. Let's dive into a world of flavors that will keep you energized, satisfied, and glowing from the inside out!

Nourishing Breakfasts

1. Chia Seed Pudding with Berry Compote

Ingredients:

- 1/4 cup chia seeds
- 1 cup unsweetened almond milk
- 1 tsp vanilla extract
- 1 cup mixed berries
- 1 tbsp maple syrup

Mix chia seeds, almond milk, and vanilla. Refrigerate overnight. In the morning, top with berry compote (berries simmered with maple syrup).

2. Green Goddess Smoothie Bowl

Ingredients:
- 1 frozen banana
- 1 cup spinach
- 1/2 avocado
- 1 tbsp almond butter
- 1 cup unsweetened almond milk
- Toppings: sliced almonds, chia seeds, fresh berries

Blend all ingredients except toppings until smooth. Pour into a bowl and add toppings.

3. Turmeric Spiced Oatmeal
Ingredients:
- 1/2 cup rolled oats
- 1 cup water

- 1/4 tsp turmeric
- 1/4 tsp cinnamon
- 1 tbsp ground flaxseed
- 1 tbsp chopped walnuts
- 1/2 sliced banana

Cook oats with water, turmeric, and cinnamon. Top with flaxseed, walnuts, and banana.

Energizing Lunches and Dinners

1. Rainbow Quinoa Bowl
Ingredients:
- 1 cup cooked quinoa

- 1 cup mixed roasted vegetables (bell peppers, zucchini, sweet potato)
- 1/4 avocado, sliced
- 2 tbsp hummus
- Handful of spinach
- 1 tbsp pumpkin seeds
Dressing: 1 tbsp olive oil, 1 tsp lemon juice, pinch of salt and pepper

Arrange all ingredients in a bowl and drizzle with dressing.

2. Lemon Herb Baked Salmon

Ingredients:
- 4 oz wild-caught salmon

- 1 tbsp olive oil
- 1 tsp dried herbs (oregano, thyme, rosemary)
- 1 lemon, sliced
- Salt and pepper to taste

Brush salmon with olive oil, sprinkle with herbs, salt, and pepper. Top with lemon slices. Bake at 400°F for 12-15 minutes.

3. Detox Veggie Stir-Fry
Ingredients:
- 1 cup mixed vegetables (broccoli, carrots, snap peas)
- 1/2 cup cooked brown rice
- 1/4 cup cooked edamame

- 1 tbsp coconut oil
- 1 clove garlic, minced
- 1 tsp grated ginger

Sauce: 1 tbsp tamari, 1 tsp sesame oil, 1 tsp rice vinegar

Stir-fry veggies in coconut oil with garlic and ginger. Add rice, edamame, and sauce. Cook until heated through.

Cleansing Smoothies and Juices

1. Green Detox Smoothie

Ingredients:

- 1 cup spinach
- 1/2 cucumber

- 1/2 green apple
- 1/2 lemon, juiced
- 1-inch piece ginger
- 1 cup coconut water

Blend all ingredients until smooth.

2. Beet Boost Juice

Ingredients:
- 1 medium beet
- 2 carrots
- 1 apple
- 1-inch piece ginger
- 1/2 lemon, juiced

Juice all ingredients and enjoy immediately.

3. Tropical Turmeric Smoothie

Ingredients:
- 1/2 cup frozen mango
- 1/2 cup frozen pineapple
- 1 banana
- 1 tsp turmeric
- 1 cup coconut milk
- 1 tbsp chia seeds

Blend all ingredients until smooth.

Healing Broths and Soups

1. Immune-Boosting Chicken Bone Broth
Ingredients:
- 2 lbs chicken bones
- 1 onion, quartered

- 2 carrots, chopped
- 2 celery stalks, chopped
- 2 cloves garlic, crushed
- 1 tbsp apple cider vinegar
- 1 bay leaf
- Water to cover

Simmer all ingredients for 12-24 hours. Strain and enjoy.

2. Detox Vegetable Soup
Ingredients:
- 1 onion, diced
- 2 cloves garlic, minced
- 2 carrots, chopped
- 2 celery stalks, chopped
- 1 cup chopped kale

- 1 can diced tomatoes
- 4 cups vegetable broth
- 1 tsp turmeric
- 1 tsp dried thyme
- Salt and pepper to taste

Sauté onion and garlic. Add remaining ingredients and simmer for 20 minutes.

3. Miso Ginger Broth

Ingredients:

- 4 cups water
- 2 tbsp white miso paste
- 1-inch piece ginger, sliced
- 1 clove garlic, crushed
- 1 handful spinach

- 1/4 cup sliced mushrooms
- 1 green onion, chopped

Simmer water with ginger and garlic for 10 minutes. Remove from heat, stir in miso. Add veggies and let sit for 2 minutes before serving.

Satisfying Snacks and Treats

1. Avocado Chocolate Mousse
Ingredients:
- 1 ripe avocado
- 2 tbsp raw cacao powder
- 2 tbsp maple syrup
- 1/4 tsp vanilla extract
- Pinch of sea salt

Blend all ingredients until smooth. Chill before serving.

2. Crunchy Roasted Chickpeas

Ingredients:
- 1 can chickpeas, drained and rinsed
- 1 tbsp olive oil
- 1 tsp cumin
- 1 tsp paprika
- 1/4 tsp salt

Toss chickpeas with oil and spices. Roast at 400°F for 20-30 minutes, shaking pan occasionally.

3. Apple Slices with Almond Butter

Ingredients:
- 1 apple, sliced
- 2 tbsp almond butter
- Sprinkle of cinnamon

Arrange apple slices on a plate. Drizzle with almond butter and sprinkle with cinnamon.

Remember, these recipes are just starting points. Feel free to experiment and adjust based on your preferences and nutritional needs. The key is to focus on whole, nutrient-dense ingredients that support your body's natural detoxification processes.

As you explore these recipes, pay attention to how different foods make you feel. This awareness is a crucial part of the Somatic Detox experience. You're not just nourishing your body – you're learning to listen to it and understand its needs.

Happy cooking, detox warrior! May your kitchen be filled with the aromas of healing foods and the joy of nourishing yourself from the inside out. Bon appétit!

Conclusion

Embracing a Lifelong Journey of Wellness

As we reach the end of this transformative journey, it's important to recognize that true wellness isn't a destination—it's a lifelong adventure. The 21-day Somatic Detox Diet you've just completed is more than a quick fix; it's a gateway to a new way of living that honors the profound connection between your body and mind.

Throughout this book, we've explored the intricate dance between physical detoxification and mental clarity. You've learned how to nourish your body with wholesome, nutrient-dense foods that support your natural cleansing processes. But more than that, you've discovered the power of mindfulness in eating, moving, and living.

Remember those first tentative steps in Week One? The gentle cleansing that seemed so challenging at first gradually became second nature. As you progressed through the deep cleansing of Week Two, you may have noticed not just physical changes, but a shift in your emotional landscape too. By Week Three, as you embraced rebalancing and rejuvenation, you likely felt a new sense of vitality and purpose.

But here's the real magic: this journey doesn't end here. The principles you've learned and the habits you've formed are tools you can carry with you for life. Your body is now primed to efficiently process nutrients and eliminate toxins. Your mind is clearer, more focused, and better equipped to handle stress. You've experienced firsthand how what you eat directly impacts how you feel and think.

As you move forward, remember that perfection isn't the goal—progress is. There will be days when you indulge, times when stress creeps back in, or moments when you fall back into old patterns. That's okay. What matters is your ability to recognize these moments and gently guide yourself back to balance using the techniques you've learned.

Consider incorporating seasonal mini-cleanses into your routine, using the recipes and meal plans provided in this book. These periodic resets can help you stay on track and reconnect with your body's innate wisdom. And don't forget the power of community—share your journey with friends and family. You might be surprised at how your positive changes inspire others.

The science is clear: a diet rich in whole, plant-based foods, combined with mindful living practices, can lead to profound improvements in both physical and mental health. From reduced inflammation and improved digestion to enhanced mood and cognitive function, the benefits of this lifestyle are far-reaching and well-documented.

As you close this book, take a moment to reflect on your progress. Celebrate the small victories and the big breakthroughs. Recognize the strength and resilience you've discovered within yourself. You've not just completed a diet; you've embraced a new way of living that honors the complex interplay between your body and mind.

Remember, wellness is not about deprivation or punishment. It's about nourishment, balance, and joy. It's about making choices that align with your highest good, while also being gentle with yourself when you stumble. You now have the knowledge and tools to make informed decisions about your health, guided by a deeper understanding of your body's needs.

So, as you step forward from here, carry with you the lessons of mindfulness, the power of whole foods, and the transformative potential of aligning your diet with your body's natural rhythms. Your 21-day journey may be complete, but your path to vibrant, holistic health is just beginning.

Here's to your continued growth, to listening to your body's wisdom, and to embracing the beautiful, ongoing journey of wellness. May each day bring you closer to the vibrant, balanced life you deserve. Your future self will thank you for the commitment you've made today. Keep nurturing your body, calming your mind, and nourishing your spirit. The best is yet to come.

If you enjoyed the content, consider sharing your experience by leaving a review. It's a great way to help others discover the book and could make a difference for those seeking similar insights. Your feedback is truly appreciated!

www.ingramcontent.com/pod-product-compliance
Lightning Source LLC
Chambersburg PA
CBHW061350250726
48657CB00004B/1417